This book belongs to

_____

This is your

fl🌸wer

For Una

This is your flower. It is the same as every other flower but this one is different because this one belongs to you. It is yours.

You may not think it is very pretty, but it is. It is a very beautiful flower and it does amazing things. Here are some things you should know about your flower...

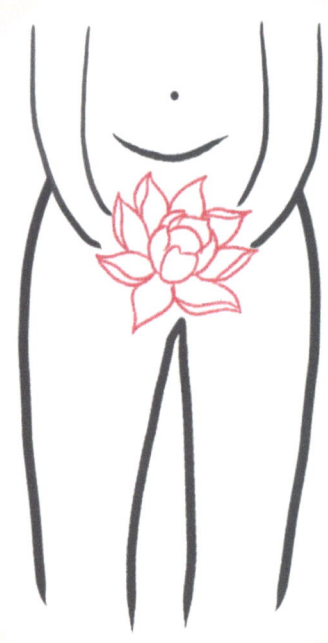

Your flower is sensitive so you must look after it. Sometimes you may notice that your flower doesn't smell as nice as it used to. That is why it's important to lightly wash it with water.

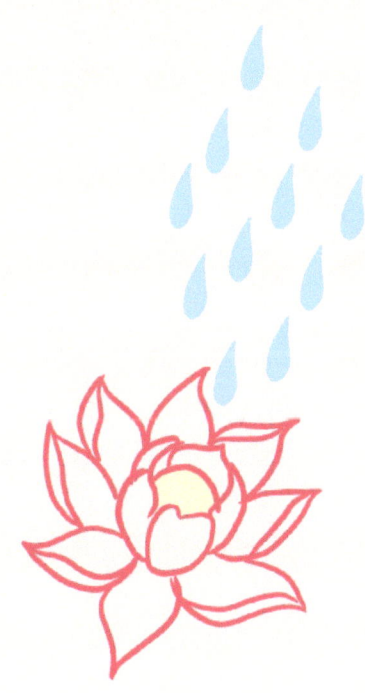

One day your flower will shed. Don't worry this happens to all little girls when they grow up. This will happen every month when it regrows.

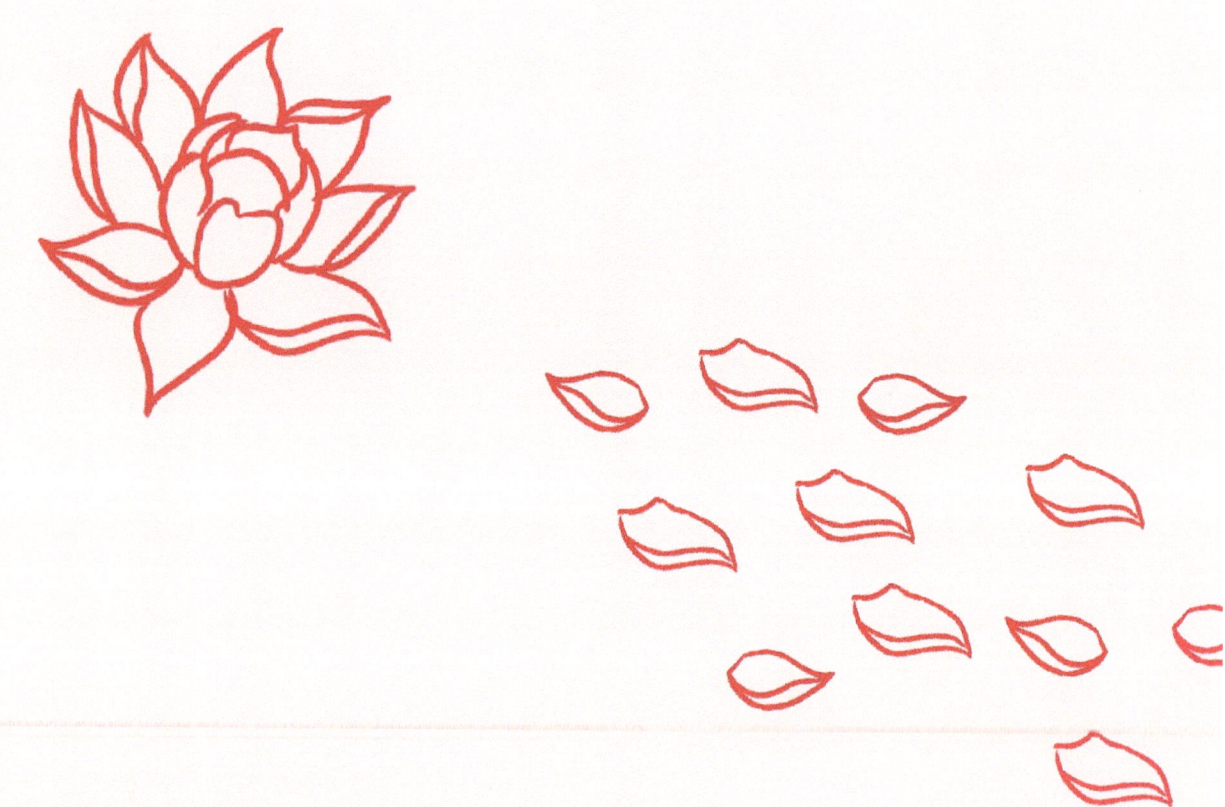

Sometimes the shedding may be heavy and sometimes it may be light. It may also hurt a little but it can also hurt a lot. This is normal. Try to make yourself comfortable at this time.

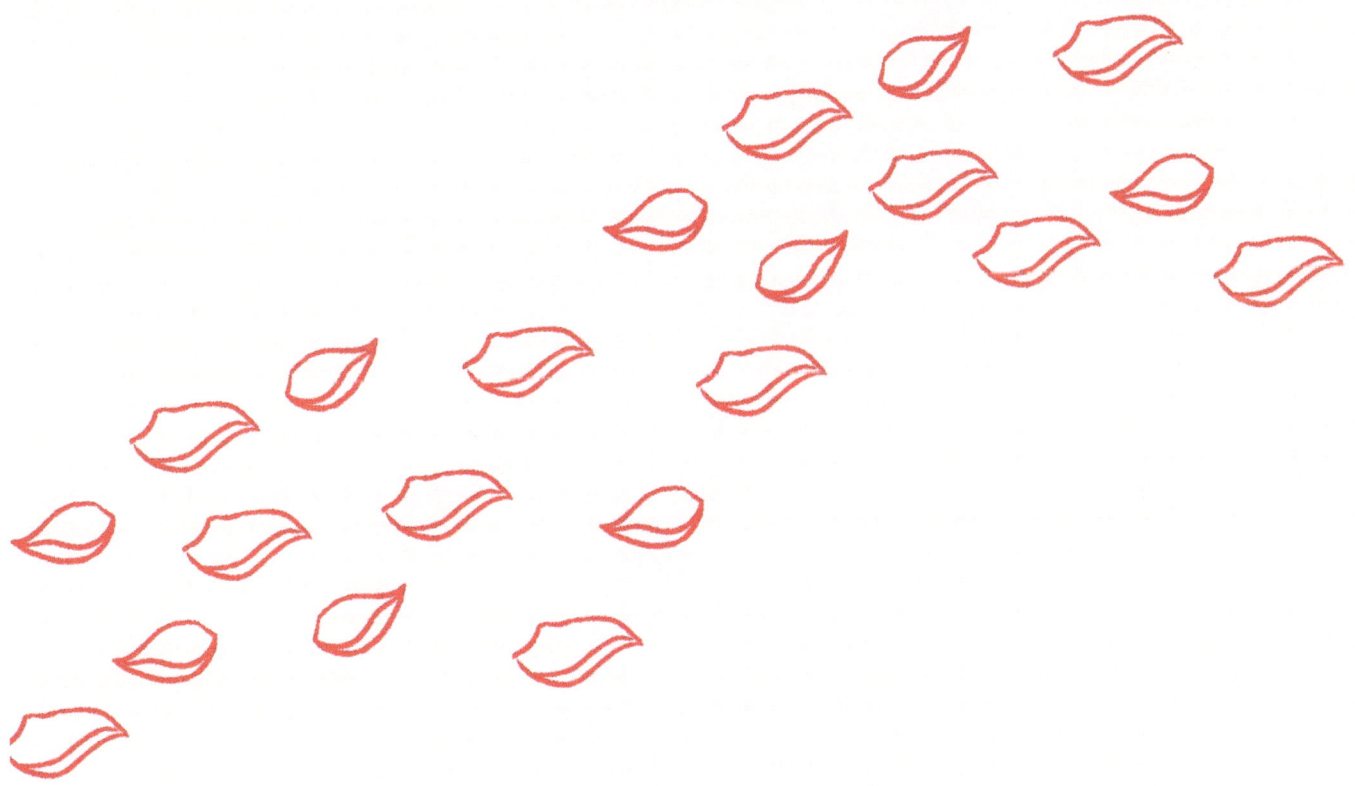

Your moods can change during this time. You might cry, you might shout, you may even go quiet for a while. It will pass. Remember this is normal too.

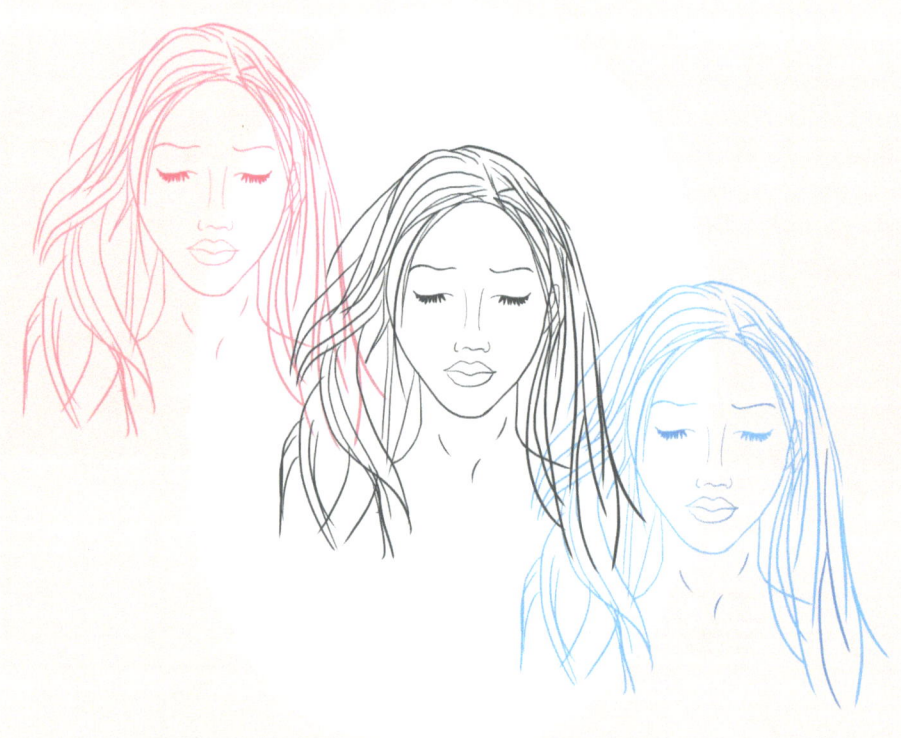

Then when you are grown and your flower is fully developed someone will want to share it with you. Remember it is your choice to let them share it. It is always your choice. It is your flower and it will always be your flower.

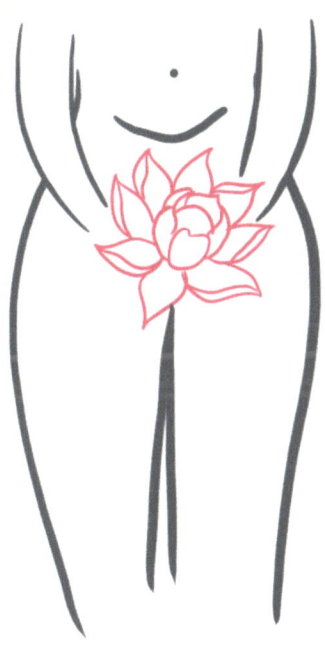

It's very important to choose wisely who you allow to share your flower because you want them to take good care of it too. If they don't, it may cause your flower problems later on.

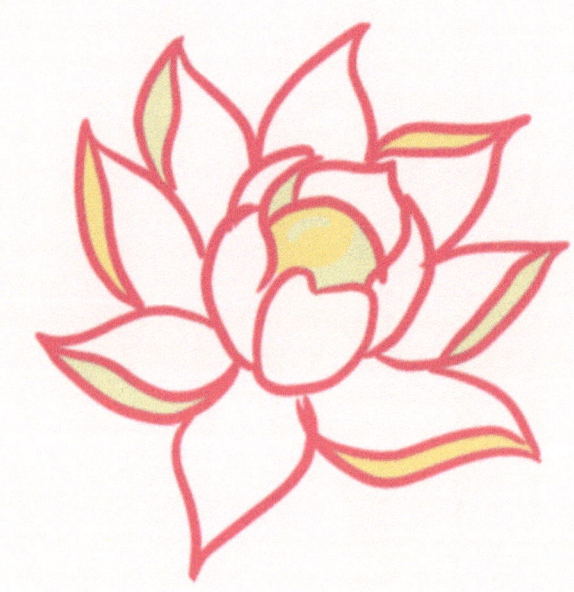

If you decide to share your flower you should know that your flower may grow a baby. This is a big responsibility and can be a very difficult situation especially when you are still very young. So think carefully about protecting your flower.

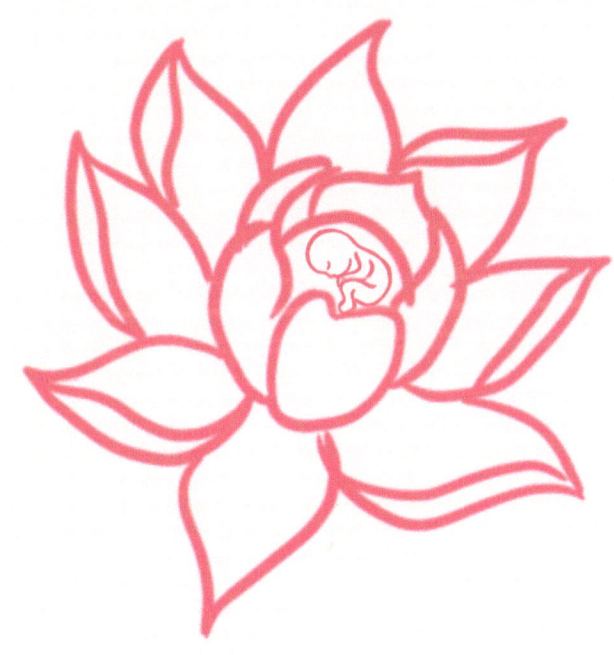

Then one final day when you are much, much older, your flower will stop shedding. It will still affect your moods and it may even cause you to feel different in many other ways too.

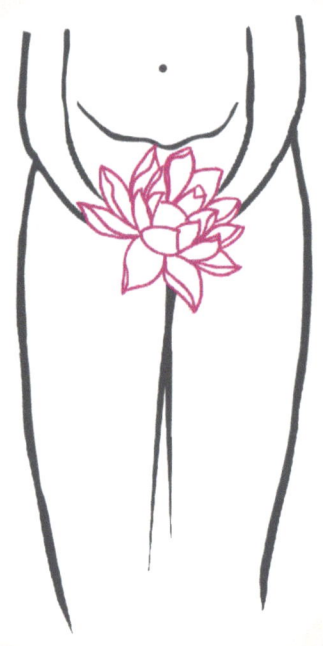

There will be days when you don't like your flower. This is normal too. You can be whoever you want to be. Remember this is your choice because this is your flower.

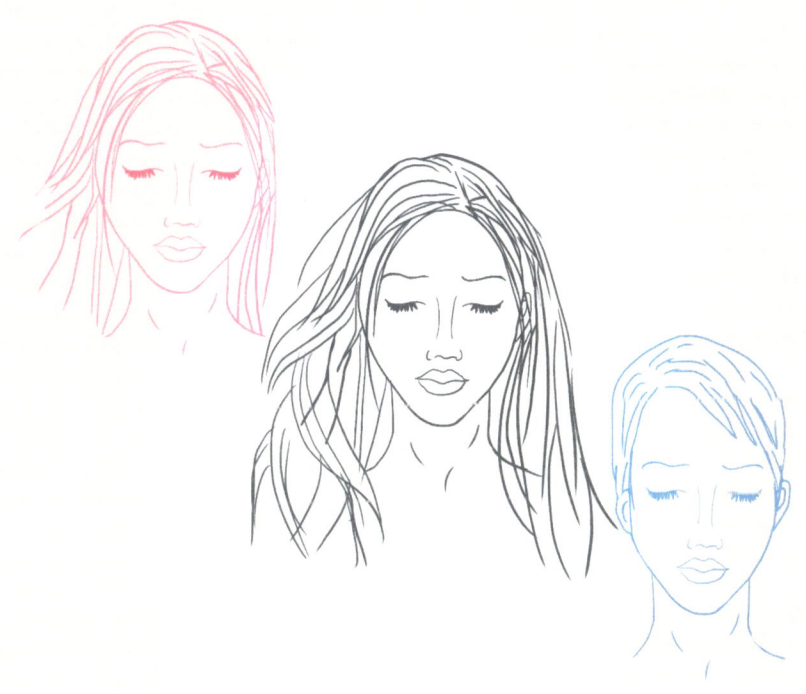

This is your flower

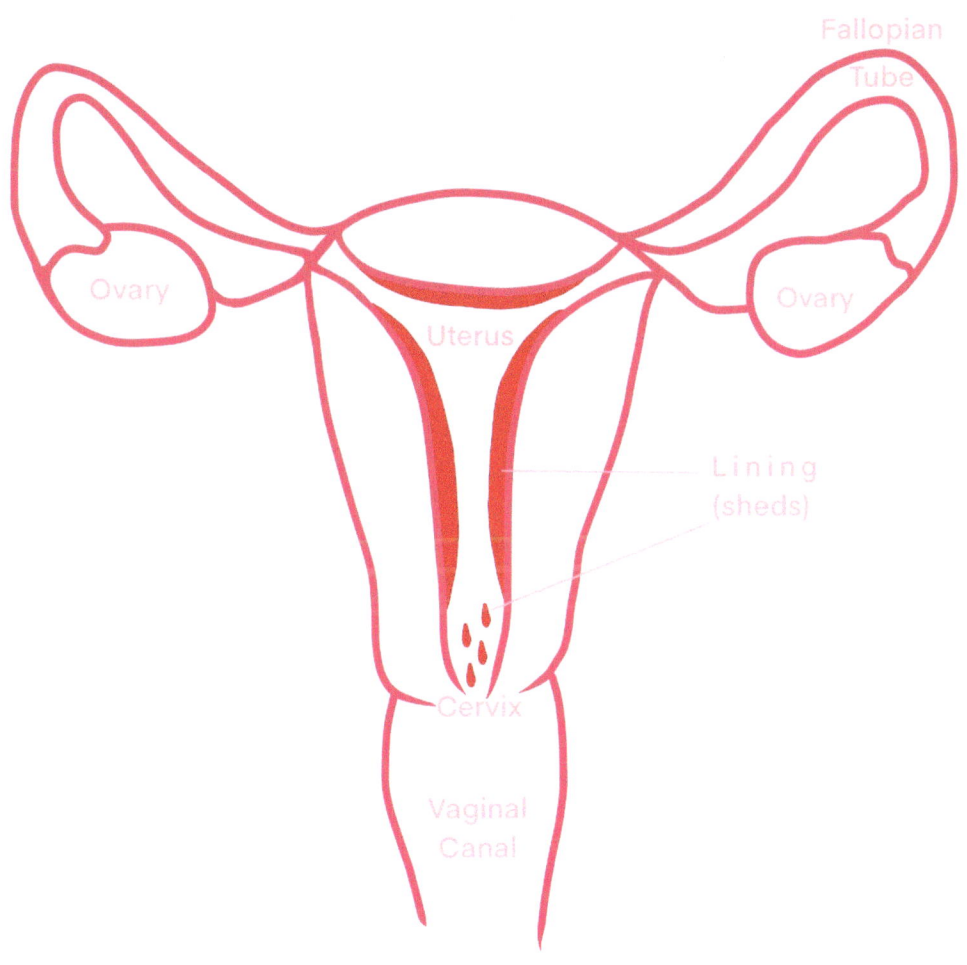

When you feel your child is ready you can replace the word 'flower' with the word 'vagina'

More books by the author available on Amazon now

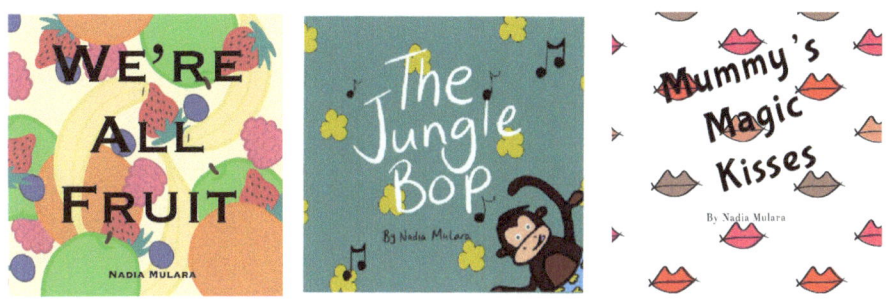

Don't forget to check out the Ocean Adventures series

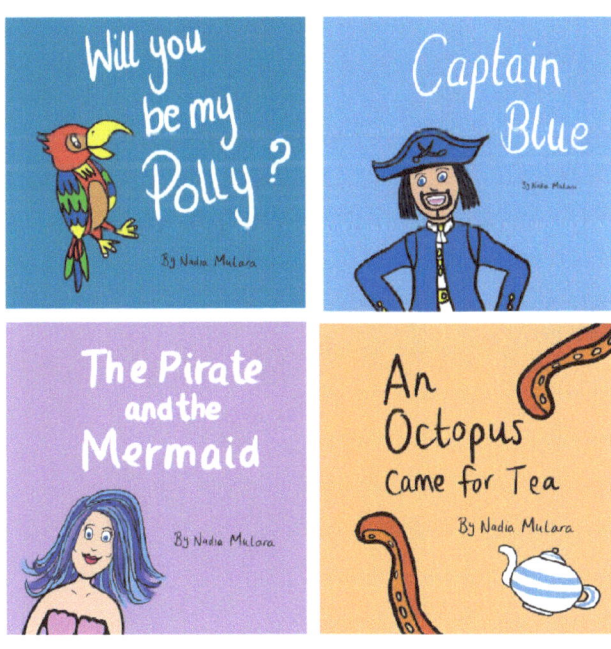

Social Media Pages

Join us online for news of upcoming competitions and new publications.

https://nadiamulara.wixsite.com/nadiamulara

Facebook

Author Nadia Mulara

Instagram

Author_nmulara

www.ingramcontent.com/pod-product-compliance
Lightning Source LLC
Chambersburg PA
CBHW060824290526
45792CB00005BB/1782